GUIDE TO
EATING OUT

**The Lick-by-Lick Guide to
Mouthwatering and Orgasmic Oral Sex**

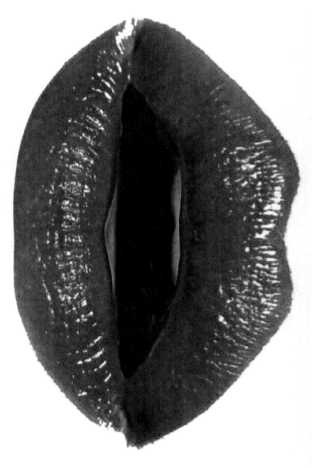

GUIDE TO
EATING OUT

The Lick-by-Lick Guide to Mouthwatering and Orgasmic Oral Sex

by
Palmer Strong

For more information on this series, please visit us on the web at
SecretLifePublishing.com

ISBN 978-0-9818039-1-3

KRE, LLC
PO Box 121135
Nashville, TN 37212-1135

Contents

Introduction

Once upon a time, men were men and, well, women – they were at home. It's not politically correct anymore, but that's the way it used to be. As men, we were the hunters, the ones off on a wild adventure to slay the beast and drag its carcass home. Time passed and, instead of hunting wild animals, men became the explorers of the world. We sailed ships and got ourselves lost on foreign continents. And the women were still at home. The women weren't necessarily happy with this but, most of the time, they were too busy raising children to really do much about it. Not only that, society taught them to accept their lot in life.

Eventually, during the Romantic Era, a change occurred. Women were no longer content to be ignored. Rather, they insisted on being courted. Marriages moved away from being a business arrangement and were destined to become a love match. Of course, this put men under a great strain. We had to learn how to prove our romantic intentions. Flowers, chocolates, serenading on balconies, and picnics by the lake – all of a sudden this became the man's domain. And what happened? Well, hey, men did it. We became the romantic love matches that women desired because, after all, we still we wanted to keep getting some action in the bedroom. Sure, it was still common to have a mistress or to visit the local working girls for those sex practices considered unsavoury in a nice romantic marriage, but we muddled through.

This seems to be where a lot of us are stuck today. We're still trying to be the romantic men the girls desire– so long as we think it will get us some action. We'll say "I Love You," or hand over the roses, but our eyes are still firmly on the bedroom. Unfortunately, women are wising up to this ploy and being a romantic isn't necessarily enough to get you what you want.

Women have changed. Yes, they still love the romance. But they are much more aware of their own bodies and their own needs. Women are entering the workforce in record numbers, delaying childhood and even delaying marriage. Not only that – today's women want sex. After years of keeping their desires to themselves, they are allowed to admit to their own sexual needs. It's true. More women now would admit to one-night stands, sexy flings and dirty weekends, then perhaps at any time in history. To some extent, women are the new men. They can call the shots and go off as explorers of the world. And, if you don't shape up, they will just leave you at home.

So, it's time to get with the program. We need to learn exactly what it is women want and learn how to give it to them. No one wants to be left out in the cold. A big part of learning what women want is learning to please them sexually. It's not such a bad thing at all – for if you can learn to please a woman in bed, then the world's your oyster. Besides, practicing will be a lot of fun!

Think of a woman's body as one of the last great unexplored continents. All of those hundreds of years we spent rampaging across the seas and we didn't stop to think about the most enjoyable unknown continent of them all – a naked woman.

You may think you already know everything there is to know about sex, but we're not talking wham, bam, thank you ma'am style sex here. We're going to talk about oral sex – cunnilingus. going down, eating out, muff diving. pussy licking, munching, grazing, growling or whatever you want to call it.

Get comfortable, this is going to be some ride.

Chapter 1: Learning About Her

Anatomy

Now, don't groan at the mention of the word anatomy. This isn't going to be some boring science class and it isn't going to involve an awful lot of grainy diagrams that make sense to no one – even the girls that are actually in possession of their own vaginas. The information I'm going to pass on to you comes from many years of hands on experience with my own lovers – and, yes, the pun is intended.

Before I get started, I have to touch on a very important subject: Porn. For most of us, our education on the anatomy of a woman comes from looking at pictures in men's magazine or surfing the web for porn. I want to tell you right up front that most of the pictures you've seen of naked women do not represent

Slightly more than half of American teenagers between the ages of 15 ando 19 have engaged in oral sex, with females and males reporting similar levels of experience, according to the most comprehensive national survey of sexual behaviors ever released by the Federal government.

The report, which was released in September 2005 by the National Center for Health Statistics, shows that experience this increases with age, with about 70 percent of all 18- and 19-year-olds doing the deed.

what that woman really looks like "down there". For aesthetic reasons, as well as because of censorship laws in some countries, a woman's private parts have often been airbrushed beyond all reality. On the whole, women do not look like a coin slot. So what does a normal woman look like?

Although every woman would disagree an Italian guy by the name of Realdo Colombo claimed that he found the clitoris in the 16th century. He published a book called *De re anatomica*, where he described it as the "seat of woman's delight." Columbo also decided that he was some sort of genius that was deserving of honor and glory. He was reported to have said, "Since no one has discerned these projections and their workings, if it is permissible to give names to things discovered by me, it should be called "The love or sweetness of Venus."

Road Map

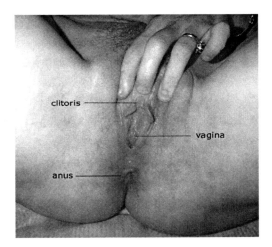

clitoris

vagina

anus

"My old boyfriend could never find my clit. Once, in frustration, I spread my legs and placed a CD on myself – with the hole over the right area. He got the message."
Jesse, 19

Innie vs Outies

You'd be wrong if you thought only belly buttons had the option of being innies or outies. It's possible for vaginas to appear neatly packaged and similar to the coin slot mentioned above, but it's not always the case. There are two types of lips on a vagina and the inner lips can actually extend way out past the outer lips. Not only that, but the rest of the vagina can also be tucked away out of sight. The vagina may also look like it's just exploded, with everything, including the clitoris – almost on public display. It's usually these "outie" types that you wouldn't see in mainstream magazines. You have to feel sorry for girls who grow up thinking they are not normal. Women can become self-conscious of their lips, so don't freak out if you take a lady home and she strips for you and you

Only once in my life have I been injured by orgasm. I'm not sure exactly what technique my lover was using, but I came so hard that I nearly kicked him with a strong leg cramp. When it was all over though, I still felt a little weird "down there." I thought maybe he'd just been a bit rough or grazed me with his teeth. But a day or so went by and it still hurt. I eventually got a mirror and found that one of my inner lips were swollen! I had to go to the doctor. Somehow, I'd got so engorged with the blood flow leading up to orgasm that some of the blood was trapped in one lip. Very odd. Nothing to do but wait it out really. It did fix itself, except now I swear that the lip on that side of my body is permanently a bit longer and floppier now.

Laura, 32

notice something dangling between her legs. It is actually quite common. As far as I know, no research has been done on the issue, but from the lovers I've had, I'd estimate that perhaps nearly a third of women have outies to some extent.

In fact, women have been made to feel so bad about what they consider their "misshapen" bits that there is even a type of cosmetic surgery offered to shorten the lips! Insane, I say.

> *I have an outie. I try so hard not to be ashamed off it. I've heard its common in women of Eastern European decent, but I have no idea. My inner lips stretch outside my outer lips and they join. Unless I'm turned on it's almost like they are fused. It can be hard for a man to get access to the inside. So I have to pull them apart for sex. Or, if he's clever he just waits unless I'm wet and ready and they open right up. Even my clit is almost on the outside. On a bad day I joke about being an exploded cauliflower. But, with the right lover, there are all sorts of fun things to try. Like sucking and pulling on my outie bits – like a modified male head job. And I've heard there is even a fetish group for men who love women with outies.*
>
> Tam, 26

It's also not unusual for women to appear a bit "lopsided." This can sometimes be caused by injury, but it can also be natural. The same is true with breasts, which are usually lopsided and they may even be different sizes. This little piece of information will certainly get you looking closely at your lover's breasts the next time she's naked in front of you. If you ask her, she will probably even be able to tell you which one is bigger or which one sets higher on her chest.

Pubic Hair

Pubic hair naturally comes in all sizes, shapes, and colors. So, as a man wanting to impress a woman in the bedroom, you'll have to get used to it. Of course, black is the most common color, but there will find all kids of shades – ranging from mousy blonde/brown to red. Yes, the ol' firecrotch. Sometimes, you can guess the color of the pubic hair just by looking at the coloring of the girl. Still, it wouldn't be wise to express your surprise at what you see. For example, if you pick up a wonderful natural red head, you are shouldn't make a comment if her pubes aren't red. Girls don't want to hear about it.

You will also find that some hair is really thick, some is thin and some is almost patchy. Some hair is long and almost straight, while some is poodle-curly. All of these variations are perfectly normal. What you may not know is that pubic hair also spreads depending on a woman's cultural background and age. I once dated a girl who, if she didn't trim, would end up with hair that reached a good few inches down each thigh. You may also notice some girls, especially those from Mediterranean backgrounds that may even have a "snail-trail" toward their belly button. It DOES not mean they were once a man! Flip your girl over and in some cases you'll even see a slightly hairy lower back! Still normal.

Just like men, women have hair all the way around their private parts, right up to the end of their butt crack. It can be much denser and thicker in some areas, so it may take you longer to notice.

Now that you may be prepared for the hairiest of all situations, it's only logical to talk about waxing, shaving and trimming. Generally, a girl will decide on her preferred hair status long before you get with her. Luckily, not many stay au-natural. Although that is a problem if you LIKE it that way – and some men do. Mostly though, you'll have to make do with whatever you get.

The most basic option is the girl who hasn't shaved or waxed at all, but trims her hair instead. In this case, she'll have all of her natural hair but the visible patch on top will be short. From there, you'll find women who shave or wax their "bikini" line, which is the crease on their thigh, in order to keep things a bit more trim. After that, you move in toward the "landing strip" look, which is usually a completely waxed pussy except for a remaining strip of hair. And then, of course, there is the Brazilian, which is the bald eagle look. Only with the Brazilian wax does the hair from the actual vaginal lips and butt crack also come off. The other styles tend to be more about appearances and you may still find yourself getting a mouthful of hair when you go down.

Things That Can Result From Body Maintenance

If a girl waxes and you take her to bed soon after, you may notice her skin is red and may be bumpy. Most likely, the girl will be embarrassed so you shouldn't mention it. In fact, she may not have intended sex that night, so just consider yourself lucky to be getting some action. Waxing is usually something planned for sexless days because of the irritation it can cause!

Shaving can also lead to all sorts of other nasty problems, such as ingrown hairs or a dry, scaly looking shaving rash. Any sort of moisturizer will help with the shaving rash if it's too unbearable to look at, but your woman may not appreciate having an ingrown hair pointed out. After all, these pussy pimples can be quite large and may be embarrassing to the girl. These pimples won't harm you, so if you stumble upon one, just turn the lights out and don't put your mouth or tongue on that little spot! Of course you could always suggest a shower and scrub her down. Not only can this be quite sensual, it may also dislodge the stubborn hair and release the ugliness.

There is another issue that should be mentioned that can look like some sort of rash brought on by body maintenance but is actually much, much, MUCH (do you get the point) more of a delicate issue.. If you throw away your airbrushed porn magazines and actually look at the anatomy of a female's thigh, you will notice something quite curious: they have little pockets of fat at the top of each thigh, just before you get to the fun parts. These pockets are there to help protect the goods and, ironically, they can be the most sensitive spot on some women! Yes, fat can be sexy. Try kissing the pockets and see what I mean. On women of all sizes, these pockets of fat can rub together during the day. This is particularly true if the lady in question is wearing a dress or skirt. After a hard day at work or after going out for a night of dancing, this rubbing can cause a type of sweat rash. The only way to cure it is to keep the area dry and to stop the rubbing. That means being naked with your legs spread open is the ideal solution! So, offer to help a lady with this issue today!

Nasty Things No One Wants To Talk About

Yes, what I'm about to discuss is horrid. But pay attention. If you can master dealing with the issues below, you can pretty much guarantee access to any woman at any time. Don't screw up your face and listen without making gagging noises, okay?

Thrush

From what I've learned, thrush is probably the worst thing about being a woman. It's a yeast infection and can be inside the vagina and on the outside of the vulva – all over those lovely lips you want to play with. This is probably one of the only times you will have absolutely no chance of going down. The woman will be itchy and sore. She may even be red and swollen. She may have a discharge that can even, believe it or not, be chunky! It'll be white or yellow and quite thick. Most women will know they have thrush and warn you – but if you ever spot these symptoms you really need to let her know so she can be treated. Treatment, which is usually a cream or vaginal pessary, can take a few days to work. So, you may be out of luck for awhile. It's also probably the best weapon a woman has to turn you down and be nasty about it. Say you're in a bar and you think all is going well and the woman turns to you and says she has a yeast infection. That's one MEAN brush off that is designed to repulse you. So, walk away. If she is interested, but *actually* does have thrush, she would have come up with other ideas – such as giving you a blow job at least!

Her Period

For the hygienically minded woman, and the game guy, periods are by no means the end of oral sex. Quite simply the woman can keep a tampon in place and, so long as there is no leakage from the tampon, the rest of her vagina is will still be fair game and blood free. Most women aren't turned on by oral sex during their periods because sometimes they can be too sensitive, or feel too crampy. But studies show that orgasms can help period pain, so try that as a pick up line. Or at least offer to give her a massage and a heat pack. Be extra gentle and you may find yourself in the driver's seat after all – because for a small percentage of women, they actually feel extra sexy during their periods! It's a hard situation to judge, but you can give it your best shot. Just like with thrush though, the mention of this condition in the bar usually means you've getting the brush off. Sorry.

"I have never had a lover that was keen on oral sex while I had my period. Then I had a fling with this one guy. He seemed normal enough and we had a great couple of weeks of late night booty calls. Then, one night he wanted to come over and I told him that I had my period so maybe we should forget it! But he was there in a flash. He put a couple of towels on the bed and asked me to have a quick shower but not change my tampon. I get horny when I do have my period so I was pretty excited – and nervous. Then he threw me down on the bed and started to go down on me. As I was getting in to it he pulled out my tampon and flung it across the room! I nearly died of shock. Then he started using his fingers inside me, painting my thighs too with the blood. I was a bit numb. It was an experience I guess, not sure I'd do it again. Thank goodness for the towels though!"

Louise, 25

Ovulation

You probably wonder why you should care about ovulation. Well the obvious thing is this – hopefully if you're having more than just oral sex, you're being safe and don't want to get the girl pregnant! But it's far more than that. Ovulation occurs about 14 days after the first day a girl starts bleeding each month. Her body changes and so do her secretions! So, if you are going down on a girl, you may find her smell is much stronger and her mucus is much thicker! If this worries you, then stick more to her clitoris than any other part of her– but we'll cover that later. There is a great side effect of this process.

For some women, they are totally, totally, UP FOR IT. I mean it's nature's way of trying to get them sperminated at their most fertile. But you can use that to your advantage – although you may just be pinned down and jumped on anyway because, for some women, it's the closest thing to becoming a wild animal you'll ever see.

This happened to me once on a day when I wasn't even looking to pick up some action. I was just having a latte after work when a woman pulled up a seat next to me. She offered to buy me another and I swear it wasn't half an hour before we were in a cab and on our way back to her place. After a few hours of great sex, she finally told me that it was her time of the month – not her period, but ovulation.

This ovulation horniness can last a few days – three or four at most. There will be a lead up period to the sexiest day and then a deflation of her horniness afterward. After that, her body will start to prepare for her next period and she may start to feel a lower pain threshold, lower tolerance of emotions, mood swings, anger, cravings and sore breasts. So this time is a great time to play very, very gentle in the bedroom.

It's Not Always Pink Down There

A girls' private parts are not always the bright glossy pink you're lead to imagine. Usually, the skin color is slightly darker than the rest of the gal's body. So, if you're taking home a beautiful caramel-skinned supermodel (and haven't we all wanted to do that at one time or another) don't be too alarmed to see she's very dark down there. That's normal. Even on white girls, the vulva can appear a light brown. And the color can change depending on blood supply and arousal. I'm not talking like some drastic change from pink to yellow or anything crazy, but a slight reddening of the pussy isn't a bad thing. You do need to keep your wits about you though if the area seems to be a bright red kind color. Then you may be looking at a case of thrush, as mentioned above. There is even a crazy infection that can turn a girl's pussy white, or very, very pale. If you see something totally out of the ordinary like that then let the lady know! The only other freaky thing you may see is basically a Michael Jackson influenced vagina. As in, it's got vitiligo. That condition can appear on any part of the body, or even just in the vagina, and results in patchy areas of skin that may be white because there area doesn't have normal skin pigment. It's not a health issue. Nd it can be treated, but most girls probably wouldn't bother unless it was on prominent areas of skin like on the arms or face.

Piercings

It's probably a good idea to get a handle on whether or not the woman of your dreams (or at least this Friday night) is wearing any metal where you can't see it. You don't want to go fumbling in the area without preparation if that's the case.

There are a few types of vaginal piercings that your lady may have. The most common piercing is a ring or bar that goes through the hood of the clitoris. It can also be in either a vertical or horizontal position. It's very rare for anyone to pierce the actual clitoris. So, she tells you it's a "clit piercing" she probably means it's sitting between her legs over the clitoris and through the hood. This can be gently tugged on and any action taking place between the legs will also make the ring rub the clit and create arousal.

After hood piercing, inner labia piercings are the next most popular choice. Since the lips can be of varying lengths, this piercing could potentially go through an extremely fleshy and visible part of her body. Inner labia piercings can be just as sexually stimulating than other types of piercings.

The outer lips can also be pierced but this is usually just for visual effect rather than for sexual stimulation.

I once had a lover who thought it would be a great idea to get his tongue pierced to help in our oral sex. I was open about the whole idea, a bit curious. It took a week or so before he felt confident enough to start using the tongue. We were in a 69er position and it felt amazing – the extra pressure from the metal was great. I had a great big orgasm and went to move off his face. But I couldn't! Somehow my pubic hair had wrapped itself around the base of the tongue piercing. He screamed when I tried to move, and I screamed too, because I was so sensitive from my orgasm and wanted his tongue to stop moving. Eventually, after a lot of squirming, he just had to grab his piecing with his hand and yank his face away. I lost a few hairs and boy did that sting. But he was so embarrassed about it.

Julia, 22

Don't forget to also consider your own piercing when thinking about oral sex. If you have your tongue pierced, it can be a real treat for the ladies. You can even get vibrating parts for your tongue piercing – just imagine how much she will love that!

Hygiene

It's a good idea to know what is normal and what is not normal when going down on a woman. You may be surprised that women themselves are not always the best judges of their own hygiene! I mean, think about the logistics – is a woman going to bend over herself like some curious dog to sniff her own pussy? Probably not. And, unless she's examining herself with a hand mirror, she probably won't ever see the view you get. Even if the lovely lady in question showers often, she could still have hygiene problems.

> Cunnilingus has a revered place in Chinese Taoism. This is because the aim of Taoism is to achieve immortality, or at least longevity, and the loss of semen, vaginal, and other bodily liquids is believed to bring about a corresponding loss of vitality. Conversely, by ingesting the secretions from the vagina, a male or female can conserve and increase his/her chi, or original vital breath.

The first issue that can cause hygiene issues is the direction she wipes after using the toilet. If she is wiping back to front, which is a no-no (although secretly most women do it anyhow), then she could be wiping bits of poo forward to her lips. Not fun. In fact, this is one of the potential causes of thrush.

If she's pushing too hard or using low quality toilet paper, she may also leave bits of balled up toilet paper behind. Tampons can also shed some cotton, so don't be surprised if you find this left over residue as well.

If you've been out drinking and the woman has been peeing up a storm, chances are she will taste and smell slightly of urine as well.

None of this is good. The problems tend to be worse the longer and denser the public hair is – which is the downside of the shaving and waxing hassle.

But take it from me, I learned through an encounter with a sexy woman called Marie that, no mater how sexy someone can be and no matter how horny you may be, sometimes you still need to pull back. We'd gone home together and once we got naked, boy, did I see some horrid things down there!

The obvious solution is to suggest a shower. This can be sexy, even for a one-night stand. Try not to make is obvious that you're worried about her smell or taste because she might get stage fright. Make it about yourself – you could even claim to be a bit smelly, cause face it, you may well be.

Sometimes, even a shower doesn't solve the hygiene problem. Between the inner and outer lips it's possible to get a build-up of smegma – just like guys get. Unless the girl is washing carefully she may miss this. Some gals have probably never noticed but, if you see a thick white paste like substance hiding behind the inner lips, you'll know what it is. It's not dangerous, but it figuring out how to let the girl know about it can be! She may be clueless, so try getting in the shower with her and trying some foreplay with your fingers. It should solve the problem if you're "handy"!

STDs

There isn't much to know about oral sex and sexually transmitted diseases when it comes to the woman's anatomy. But, if you have a cold sore, you can't go down on a woman unless you're an utter bastard who doesn't care about the woman's health! You can give her genital warts this way and it's an STD with NO CURE. It works the opposite way too – if you see warts on her, then you must not perform oral sex. Warts can look round and flat they can be found in groups or alone, or then can be small or large. Since they are painless, she may not even know she has them. Sorry dude, but it's your job to tell her if you see them!

Having said that, oral sex can expose you to the same types of risks as any type of sex. Chlamydia, gonorrhea, herpes, hepatitis (multiple strains), and HIV — they can be transmitted through oral sex. The risk may be lower than penetrative sex, but it is still there. You will increase the chances of contracting something if you have any cuts on your face, mouth, lips or gums. So, if in doubt, then call off the hot and heavy sex session.

For extra protection, you might want to consider using dental dams. Most sex shops will sell them or you can make your own by cutting a condom up one side to make a square bit of latex and placing it in your mouth with the lubed side down. It isn't great to taste latex, but it will give you some idea of how a woman feels giving head to a guy wearing a condom.

Aging

A section on anatomy wouldn't be complete without a mention of the effects of aging. I mean, there are plenty of MILFs, and even GILFs, out there on the scene. And the phenomenon of the "cougar," or older woman hunting for younger men, is a great thing for us that like to play. Now, plastic surgery may have fixed most things on your babe, but you will notice her private areas are softer and not as "solid" as those of a younger girl. Gravity may have pulled and stretched things. Changes in hormones may have weakened muscles. There may be wrinkles and grey

> When I was in my early 20's, I met my first cougar. I have always considered myself experienced, but what she showed me in that one night blew my mind. Whatever she thought she lacked in appearance or age she made up in experience. She taught me several of my best oral tricks that I still use today!

pubic hair too. You might also have to work extra hard to identify exactly how to turn her on if her clitoral hood has slipped or is sagging too much over her clitoris. She might also have a problem with dryness – so lube may be essential! But none of these issues are major and, with a little extra work, the rewards are all yours! Hello, Sugar Mama!

Childbirth

There are plenty of Yummy Mommies out there. Childbirth may have changed their anatomy slightly, but you may not even notice a difference! During penetration, you may notice that the woman feels looser, but this is more an urban myth than reality and only a small minority of women will feel this way. Really, the vast majority of women will feel exactly the same as pre-birth. After all, the vagina is designed to deliver babies and repair itself!

If you have a particularly giving lover that is happy to let you look at her closely, you may notice a scar running from the base of her vagina toward her anus. This could be the result of either a doctor cutting the area in order to allow a baby's head to pass or it could be the result of a doctor having to repair natural tearing that happened during childbirth. This should not, however, have an impact on your love life.

The other scar you may see will be located on the top of her mound at the panty line. This is a sign that she had a caesarean delivery. Usually, this scar will run horizontally, though it can be vertical instead.

There is one other thing that should be mentioned about childbirth. The pressure of delivering a baby can leave the woman slightly incontinent. That is, she may leak urine if she laughs, sneezes, picks up something heavy or jumps. This is an acutely embarrassing problem for some women. So, if she won't allow you to go down on her but won't say exactly why, chances are she's not sure it's safe for you!

Chapter 2: It's All In the Technique

Now that you have the anatomy basics down, you will no longer be surprised by anything you see and you'll know how to identify the parts of a normal, healthy woman. You'll also know what the unhealthy, unhygienic issues can be and their

> The term for oral sex comes from an alternative Latin word for the vulva *(cunnus)* and from the Latin word for tongue *(lingua)*. A person who performs cunnilingus may be referred to as a "cunnilinguist"

causes. That means you're ready to rumble. What do you actually do now? It looks like it's time to talk technique

The Basics

So, you have a tongue. The issue is – how do you use it? First, think about the different surface areas of your tongue such as the tip if you poke it out and the he top surface you use when licking an ice cream. Those are the two main areas to focus on with your tongue. Using the side of your tongue, or trying to use the underneath part of your tongue in some clever, backward-licking motion is really all too complicated and won't get you the results you want.

The tip

Using the tip of the tongue is probably the quickest way to lead a girl to orgasm. Place the tip of your tongue close to her clitoris. You can try directly on the clitoris, or the hood, but sometimes you'll need to cover the whole small area in that vicinity to ensure you don't get too intense. Don't start right on the clitoris with a lot of pressure though. You will need to warm up the girl with some all over lapping first! When she is turned on, move that tip around. Try up and down mini-strokes, and side to side. Try tracing a shape like a circle. Vary it a little without actually moving the tongue tip to a different area. Start slowly and use a fairly light, even pressure. This will help you warm up your woman and she should start to relax and maybe open her legs a bit more. You may also feel her clitoris become enlarged and engorged with blood. This is all a very positive reaction.

Now that you have reached this state, you can increase the pressure or the rhythm of the strokes you apply with the tip of your tongue. Speed up the circle pattern and the movements. In many cases, this technique is what will help a girl reach orgasm quickly and simply – and all you are using is your tongue and stimulating her clitoral area!

Call this the consistent orgasm technique 101. I have had success with this most basic of methods more times than I can count. Sometimes, I think this is the best way to approach any new lover – and then see how it goes from there.

If this method does not seem to be leading anywhere and if your lover is not relaxing and the clitoris is not enlarging and emerging from under its hood, it may be that the pressure and movement is still too intense and that the tip of your tongue is annoying her that than turning her on. So it could be time to bring out the next method.

The surface of your tongue

It's hard to control the surface area of your tongue and its position, but the effort is worth it. Think of your favorite ice cream and how you can lick with the entire surface area of your tongue from base to tip. You can apply this method when going down by using the entire surface area to lick from the vagina up to the clitoris. This method may increase her general level of arousal, but be aware that your taste buds will go into overdrive with this method and the area around the vagina will taste different from the area around the clitoris. If you are worried about this, it's best to stick with a small area of surface usage up and around the clitoral area. Bathe the area with your tongue rather than using the tip.

The surprise tip

There is, of course, a very different usage for your tongue. This method may take your lover by surprise, so don't start out with this technique. Rather, it's best used when she is already half way on her journey to orgasm. For the surprise tip technique, use your tip to penetrate her vagina. If you have a fairly flexible tongue, you can reach a good inch or so inside her, which is plenty because most of the nerve endings in the vagina are found in the first inch anyway. Using this technique shows you are not afraid of doing whatever it takes to please your lover and totally devouring her. It's best used in combination with the tip of the tongue on the clitoris, followed by a bit of surface licking and then the penetration.

If there is one thing I've learned, it is to not use this technique every time. I've used this technique during those times when the passion was so intense that I intuitively knew using my tongue in this way was going to bring on a huge orgasm, such as after being separated for a week. But, there were also times when subtle techniques were better and this technique would have been too much, such as when with a new lover and getting to know each other.

Your teeth

Latin lovers are meant to be the best, right? That's what I'd heard. So, I was so excited to meet a Venezuelan guy at a night club. He was so sexy and seductive. I was so turned on and couldn't wait to get him in bed and I was happy to let him munch on me too! But it all went horribly wrong. Granted, we were a bit drunk, but he was all teeth. Like some wildcat. He didn't hurt me, but it was the most annoying sensation in the world. He'd almost get it right with the tongue and then BAM. More teeth grazing. I faked an orgasm and then faked sleep. And thank god he left! Serves me right for believing in stereotypes I guess.

Zara, 36

Um, think about the times a girl has got a bit toothy with your penis. What did you think of the whole situation? Okay, then you pretty much can figure out the issue with teeth and going down on a woman. They are mostly a no-no. The only exception to this rule that I've ever seen is when a lover was really turned on and then I gently picked up her swollen clit with my teeth. And I mean gently.

Stubble

While we're on the topic of painful things to do, I just thought I'd mention stubble. Designer stubble can look great, worn out and about town. But it may cause issues in the bedroom later if you are too rough, or move too quickly. You would not like your penis sandpapered, so try to keep the same consideration in mind. No sudden rough movements please!

Sucking

If you have warmed up your woman with some licking and flicking of your tongue, then it is probably a fine time to start to suck gently. You could try sucking on her inner lips if they are long enough. Otherwise, the clitoris is probably enlarged enough to feel like a small marble or pea in your mouth. You can try rolling this around gently, but always listen for cues from your lover as to whether or not she finds this enjoyable. If, at any stage, she tries to pull herself away from you, it means the feeling is too intense and you should stop sucking and go back to some gentle tonguing.

Penetration

Should oral sex involve penetration? Oh yes. Does that actually mean your penis? Not likely. Penetration, for the majority of women, increases the intensity and pleasure of oral sex at least ten-fold. The trick for us men in this situation is to figure out exactly when to introduce it and how.

Let's start with the when. It should never be first. A woman needs time to get turned on and produce lubrication. Actual penetration itself isn't that arousing to a woman, because there aren't any nerve endings deep in the vagina. Most women will only have an orgasm with clitoral stimulation of some sort.

Penetration should come once you have worked your way through the licking, sucking and tonguing techniques, as advertised above. Usually, once penetration starts, orgasm is only minutes away!

Now comes the how. Think like a lesbian. They don't have a penis, so what do you think they rely on? That's right. Fingers.

Fingers are the perfect size and length to really please a woman. You will have to look at the size of your hands and figure out some basic math. Women can easily slip up to three or four fingers inside their lover, forming a kind of "duck-bill" shape to introduce a sense of deep penetration. But our hands are not delicate or flexible enough. Start with one, and then aim for two fingers. You can always ask your lover if she'd like more or less.

Don't push your fingers in quickly and start thrusting away. This may actually hurt. Besides, you're trying to multitask by keeping the tongue going as well, which will be difficult if you are jamming your fingers in her. Try just moving your fingers around slightly and wiggle them around. Or, try moving them only a little back and forward. If all of this seems to be working well, then try a few deeper or harder thrusts.

G-Spot

According to recent research, some women do have a G spot. The G spot is an area of spongy tissue located on the front wall of the vagina between the vagina and the urethra. Pressure on this area can induce huge orgasms. Hunting for the G spot has always been a good sport and, with science to back you up now, you should join in the hunt. The perfect time to explore is while your lover is close to orgasm from your tongue technique and finger penetration. Try to bend your fingers up, toward the front of your lover. You shouldn't do this when you are deep inside her, but when you are only about an inch or two inside. You can always try running your fingers along her front vaginal wall from front to back as well. Watch for her body to change its movement to know if you have found the right area. It should feel a little fleshier than the rest of the wall when you do find it and will be coin sized.

If you are man enough to have found this point, then massage it gently and push around the area. Then, watch the fireworks explode! I can speak from experience about the fireworks that the G-spot can provide. I was in bed with a lady I'd slept with a few times and I decided to go exploring for the G-spot. It was obvious I found it because she started to moan and buck like crazy. But, as soon as I took my fingers from the area, her arousal level would drop. So, of course, I kept my fingers moving there.

Eye contact

Hopefully, if you've followed the steps above in roughly the order listed, you have been successful in helping your lover reach orgasm. I just thought I should throw in a word of warning about one of the most common beginning muff-diving traps – forgetting to use your eyes or using them too much! This is probably not an obvious sex tip, but one that I know from experience to be important.

Don't just be focussed on the clitoris and peer intently into her private region. Every now and then, try to look up to her face as well. If she has her eyes open and you make eye-contact then she will think you are a gentleman who is checking in with "her mind/soul" in order to make sure she is okay. It also looks like you are gauging her reaction and she'll think that is wonderful. In actuality, it will probably also turn you on to see her panting and groaning. Just don't overdo it! Don't stare at her. She'll think you are crazy, and she'll feel under pressure to perform!

Blowing air

Another safety tip involves blowing air. Not only is this tip something that will keep your woman safe from death, it will keep you safe by not making you look like an idiot.

Never blow air into a woman's vagina. It could kill her. Granted, this is an extremely unlikely scenario, but still one you should know. Blowing in the vagina can introduce an embolism into her system, which can be fatal. Gently blowing across her privates is probably no big deal, but just don't huff 'n' puff into her.

Death aside, if you've heard that blowing air was some kind of sexy turn on, you are wrong. A woman would most likely just laugh if you attempted this manoeuvre.

Humming

Humming in oral sex? What a concept. In my experience, I've not actually found this to be of much use. But, there are over a billion women out there and I haven't slept with all of them, so you may find that one special girl that loves some humming.

The theory is that humming makes your lips vibrate – although this isn't as easy as it seems either. I mean, start humming right now. Are your lips moving or is the vibration kinda stuck in your throat? Try it on the back of your hand – let the humming actually move your lips. Okay, got it. Great. Well now that you're vibrating away, the theory continues. Place your vibrating lips on your lover's clitoris and she should love the sensation. You now just have to keep the humming going until orgasm, so make sure you've got some great tunes to hum!

Does this all seem a bit silly to you, or is it just me? I mean, what you've really done by teaching yourself to make your lips vibrate is to reinvent the wheel, so to speak. Or, er, the vibrator. But a real vibrator takes batteries, and can keep up that buzzing at a steady pace, for a long, long time. This makes it seem ideal for the task.

Still, if you want to prove that man can beat machine, hum away! I considered this a real challenge and, over a long afternoon at a lover's house, I finally perfected the humming routine. My lover suggested different songs to me and I tried to hum them on her clit! While it's not one of my favourite techniques, humming can, on the odd occasion work well.

Involving nipples

If the basic techniques above weren't already enough to get you confused and tripping over yourself in bed, then this last bit of technique will surely blow your mind.

So, let's recap. You've got your tongue going on your women's clit. You have perhaps two fingers inside her, searching and stroking for that G spot. Now, are you forgetting something? Yes, her nipples. Take the hand that isn't busy and reach up for her nipple. If she is already close to orgasm this can be the final treat! Gently pinch and tweak her nipple. If you already know your lover well, you may find that, with all of the other sensations swamping her, she prefers her nipple to be pinched quite hard.

Now, the final trick is to maintain all three things at once – fingers, tongue and nipple play – until she is writhing in pleasured agony.

Tools Of the Trade

If you feel that adding nipples makes you feel too much like an acrobat, then there are plenty of other ways you can achieve the same result.

If you want to reach the nipples, but find that you can't or if you can't manage the right tweaking and pinching that your lover likes, consider nipple clamps. These are pretty cheap and can be ordered online or bought at any sex shop. The basic ones aren't adjustable, so steer clear of them. You want to buy clamps that allow you to control the pinch factor. Otherwise, they may cause too much pain!

When she feels the time is right, your lover can clamp these onto herself mid oral sex. Or, you can help her set them up right at the beginning, before you head south. That way you can focus on her lower parts!

Using toys are fun in the bedroom but I find some guys don't know how to deal with them. Us gals have been friends with them since college, and almost all of my girlfriends have even given their vibrators a name – like Paulie, Mr Buzzy, Purple Avenger etc. We know that you need to wash them with warm soapy water, store them nicely, change the batteries and air them out once in a while. Guys – not so much. I had great oral sex with a guy once and he was using my dildo on me. Afterwards he dropped it on the floor where it picked up all sorts of nasties because, of course, it was wet. Then we went out for dinner and I came back to find the dog chewing on it. So, so, wrong.

Melis, 29

If it's the finger penetration that you are finding tough, consider a dildo. Yes, it would be nice if your penis was actually on your chin in this case so you could use that instead, but it's not. You can buy a dildo that attaches to your chin if that is what you really want, but you may look a bit silly! Instead, just get a run of the mill dildo to do the job. You can penetrate her with the dildo while your mouth continues to work.

If the penetration is fun for you, but you're getting sore from using your tongue, then the lazy version of oral sex may be for you! Use a vibrator on your lover's clit. You can then be free to use your fingers on her and not have to work your tongue! Though, now we're moving away from the very definition of oral sex. You can always use the vibrator and your tongue. That still keeps you in the game!

Cool It Down

If you want to experiment further with the basic techniques, try introducing different sensations by using ice in your mouth. Even ice cream will do the trick. You can also try warming aids. This way, you can play with different temperatures. There are creams and oils that you can apply that will either give a warm – almost burning/tingling – sensation to your lover's clit and surrounding area. You can start off slowly by sucking on a menthol drop and see what she thinks of that sensation when you use your menthol tongue. Just don't be rushing out to grab things like Tabasco sauce unless you have a plan of retreat if the sensation is too much!

A lover and I once bought almost one of every type of cooling or warming gel in a sex shop we'd stopped in at and, over the course of a week, we tried each one. For me personally, I find anything with menthol works the best.

❝Once, during a hot and heavy session in the shower, my lover and I decided to see what toothpaste felt like on my clit. I mean, we knew the brand we used had menthol in it. It was divine. A nice warm sensation and my clit was massive. Going down on me then was an odd thing my lover said, because I tasted like toothpaste. But from my point of view it was great. ❞

Kylie, 21

Positions

Starfish

Let's start with the basics. You lover lies on her back and you lie on your stomach in between her legs. This is a great start and helps achieve a really nice, guilt-free orgasm, as a woman does love the whole idea of being a starfish. Normally, she has to do nothing in this position and you do all the work.

There is nothing tricky about the starfish position, except making sure you

In the late 1980's, in the state of Georgia, a man was sentenced to five years in prison for engaging in oral sex in. It was with his wife, with her consent and in their home. His predicament was quite a source of amusement to other inmates.

lover is far enough up the bed to give you room to play between her legs. If that fails, you'll be in an awkward half-on, half-off the bed position. In that case, you are best off kneeling... but you'll then have to make her move down the bed to your face!

Scarfing

If your lover is already moving toward the end of the bed to meet your kneeling self, then suggest she throws her thighs over your shoulders. You'll then be supporting half of her body weight – so you might want a cushion. The benefit of this position is that it gets her pussy lined up perfectly with your mouth, which saves you you neck strain!

I find that, in my experience, women may be a little shy about throwing their legs over her lover. So, I like to reach up and grab them by the buttocks and almost playfully drag them to the end of the bed. Before they even realize it, I have their legs over my shoulders – and they never protest once I start.

Propped up

If holding you lover's body weight isn't going to work for you, then you can achieve the same results by asking her to place a pillow under her bottom. This will tilt her pelvis up toward you in the same way. This works really well if you have a larger lover because it will also reveal much more of her inner lips and clitoris.

69

69ing is, of course, every frat boy's dream. But the reality is often different from the fantasy because this can be a difficult position to pull off. The woman on top, crouching over you, is better for her because she can control the thrust of your penis into her own mouth. She may be far too out of control if you are thrusting from above. This position can lead to red faces and wobbly muscles. Try a modified side-on version of the 69 where you are both on your sides on the bed instead of in any gravity-defying position.

The real trick of this position is the orgasm issue. A woman may be concentrating hard on pleasing you, so much so that she forgets to turn herself on mentally and actually isn't enjoying it so much. And us men are likely to be so thrilled with the attention our penis is getting that we may slip up in our timing and pressure.

Attempt this on a one night stand at your own risk – if it works, well, you know the lady will be telling everyone about it for a million years. If it fails, you may well find yourself ridiculed on some web site like dontdatehim.com!

Sit on my face, please!

Done correctly, this position has the potential to be super hot for both you, and your lover. You get to feel like you are being smothered in lady-parts while watching her breasts too, which is a joy. In addition, she gets to control the moves a bit, directing herself onto you in a way that she knows will get her going!

For this position, it's great to have a bed head for the woman to hold on to. If you don't, it's not the end of the world, but she is going to have to balance herself using her thighs more and with her palms flat against the wall.

This can be a tricky thing for the woman, especially if she's not experienced at this position. Think about it from her point of view. She has to tense her legs, balance herself with her legs open, hover about your face, not over balance forward or backward, and then concentrate on her clit. At first, this may make an orgasm impossible. Practice will make perfect though!

Things to watch out for with the position are fairly obvious. You don't want your face mashed and you don't want to pull a neck muscle reaching up to her either – so you may have to use your hand on her hips to guide her to the right height. Once she is there her position may change asher arousal grows, so don't be afraid to again place your hands on her hips to motion to her to move up or down slightly.

There is something about sitting on your face that is amazing. Before I met you I was always worried about holding my weight above a guy's face. I'm glad you talked me into giving it a go. I have such a different strength of orgasm on your face. This will sound weird but it feels like my orgasms sometimes have colors or flavors. Not usually in any starfish kinda deal, but mostly when I'm on your face. The best ones are green orgasms. And I only have green orgasms in that one position.

Frances, 30

Also be careful about your lover's self-esteem in this position. If a woman is larger, or even thinks she is, she will not want to ride your face for fear of squashing you or, at the very least, looking very unattractive. Reassure her, perhaps use pillows to cushion her legs and, hopefully, sit back for the ride of your life!

Sitting up

If you fancy a bit of kinky role play, or even just a different take on the whole idea of oral sex, then have your lover sit on a straight backed chair – legs spread, high heels optional. Kneel before her and devour her. This is a domination-submission type of situation so vamp it up! Treat her like your queen.

On a practical note – a cushion will come in handy for your knees and even her back.

Shower

You'll notice that over, and over, and over, I mention showers in this book. Showers cure almost all issues with oral sex that revolve around smell, taste or objecting women! So, if you're going to be spending so much time in the shower, why not actually have sex there too? The foreplay is obvious – you are both naked and wet and perhaps you've been shaving your girlfriend or "making sure she's clean" and you notice that she's actually turned on. You could have her sit on the edge of a bathtub or you could kneel in front of her in order to munch her in the shower.

Do be prepared for a few laughs, however, while trying this position under a running shower! You are more than likely to end up with a mouth and nose full of water – more so if your lover has a full amount of pubic hair – which acts as a waterproofing device to funnel water off her vagina! She may have to experiment with different standing positions in the shower so as to stop the water from trickling down. But, if you bury yourself deep enough, it won't mater – the water will just run down your face and head without choking you!

Bunk bed

I thought I should mention this, especially for those of you that have kids or that have lovers with kids. Well, the kids need to be out of the picture for this little idea, but, oh my goodness, it can be fun.

Get your lover to sit or lay on the top bunk with her legs spread. She'll probably be at face height, which means you can walk right up to her and, still standing, give her a

" Once I had to go on a dreaded family vacation. There were no kids along but a ton of aunts and uncles as well as my parents. My lover and I were given the kids' bunkhouse as our room. I was so bummed that I couldn't sleep in the bed with him – well, it would have been a tight squeeze if I did. I claimed the top bunk. I have no idea how it started, but we ended up with him licking me out at head height from the top bunk. It was amazing. I wish I could do that everyday. It's the ultimate in lazy, comfortable access, isn't it? "

Pippa, 28

great oral sex experience without any neck cramping or kneeling issues! Bliss.

Using walls and headboards

This is another idea that builds on the basic positions. While you are on your belly with your face between your lover's legs in the starfish position, see if you can gain some traction with your feet. Headboards are ideal for this, as are walls, bed bases and posts. You can then use this traction to lightly spring off with your feet and knees, as if you are about to dive. This can add to your thrusting if you are using your fingers inside her or, at the very least, give a nice gentle swaying to the action of your lips and tongue.

If your woman likes it rough, then you can use a number of fingers inside her along with the thrusting of your body propelled by your feet to really, really, fuck her.

Orgasms

How it all begins

Women are tricky. Their sexual drive is linked to their emotions, which in turn is linked to whatever they are thinking about. Basically, no matter how good your fingers are, how soft your tongue is, and how many positions you try, a woman still has to think herself into the idea. It's not like that for us guys. We can have a bad day and have an argument with our girlfriends and still be happy enough to turn around for some bedroom activity. Not so for the ladies. So, an orgasm really begins with setting the scene. How much "scene-setting" you have to do will depend on if we're talking about a one night stand, your fling, or your wife of twenty years. I think you could safely assume that the longer you've been involved, the more effort you'll have to put in to prepare for a mind-blowing orgasm. This is an idea that will be mentioned again later, especially in the context of a long term relationship!

Types of orgasm

Let's start with a mental orgasm. You might not even think this is a type of orgasm, but think about all of those wet dreams you had as a kid. You

> In a recent *Elle* survey, two-thirds of women respondents said they usually or always climax during love-making.

weren't always actually hands-on in those dreams – it was something your mind conjured up and your body went along with the idea.

The same thing happens to women – but with less obvious results. Women can orgasm purely by dreaming and, even if they've been involved in a traumatic accident that results in paraplegia or quadriplegia, it remains possible that some women will continue to orgasm.

This should make you pretty comfortable with the idea that for all women, an orgasm is physically possible.

Approaching

It may take a while before you start to see any results from your efforts in going down. Sex isn't like the movies and women are not generally ready to start screaming within seconds. So, what signs should you look for to indicate an orgasm is about to occur? Increased breathing rate is a good sign. Noise can be a sign, depending on the woman. Starting to shift her body around, or moving her hips shows that she is warming up too. She may go red in the face, or start sweating. She will also become wetter.

The most obvious sign of an approaching orgasm is an engorged clit. It can be as much as double in size, so your tongue should be able to notice the difference. She may also start to experience muscle cramps or muscle spasms as the blood flow increases. Her legs may jiggle and twitch. She may put her hands on your head to guide you better.

This process of approaching orgasm can go on for some time and it does not mean all of a sudden you need to change what you are doing. She likes it if she is approaching orgasm, so the best thing to do is to continue to do the same thing! I repeat again. No new tricks at this stage.

Eventually, there will be an end point. It could be fireworks for her, with screaming and thrashing, or she could suddenly just fall backwards onto the bed with the twitching and spasms gone from her legs. The actual point of orgasm can be different each time, with different intensities.

Faking

Well, you might ask, if the actual orgasm can be different each time, then how on earth could I tell if a woman is faking it? The best advice I can give is that you shouldn't judge by the noise. Actresses can scream and moan with the best of them. Shy women can orgasm silently. So, it's not as easy as that. Don't judge by large movements, either. Again, the actresses can thrash about with the best of them, while your shy lover may lie silently.

Instead of judging by noise and movement, look for the body changes that cannot be manipulated. A women who is not turned on and heading toward an orgasm will not be able to enlarge her clitoris. A woman who is jerking and flailing around while wildly bucking her hips, but with no actual spasms or contractions happening in her legs, is most likely faking it. Going red in the face and sweating is also hard to fake, unless the lady in question is holding her breath.

"*I can't help it. I'm a screamer when I orgasm. It sounds totally fake. But it's not. Like, I think I should be being filmed. It is always a problem for roommates; even neighbors in our area are a bit close and can hear. Sometimes, I've even frightened my lovers because it can start so suddenly. I have to reassure them it's a good thing!*"

Larrisa, 22

You may be wondering why you should care. If she's happy enough to fake it, then perhaps your job is done, right? I'm sorry, but the answer is no, your job isn't over.

She may be faking it because she feels like she needs to give you an orgasm to make you stop going down. You may be that bad, so she'd rather you stop. Ouch.

She may also be too shy to really communicate what she needs to turn her on, which makes her feel embarrassed enough to fake it. She may be tired or upset or pissed off at you for not doing the dishes – any number of mental hurdles may have stopped her in her tracks. You might need to do a bit of detective work in order to uncover the reasons your lover is faking an orgasm. That way you can fix them. If you don't fix them, you're chances of getting another chance down there are slim to none!

Multiple

Multiple orgasms do exist, although every woman is not lucky enough to have them. Not only that, it can be a hit and miss kinda affair. So, I would never set out with the aim of giving a lover multiples. Rather, I would see it as a great reward for hard work, if it should happen.

A normal orgasm can be so powerful that a woman will refuse any more touch or tongue action. That means it is

I'll never forget you for showing me the multiple orgasm. And the only way I can have one is through oral sex and the marathon work of the man. It takes a lot of gentle and slow warm ups and a very good understanding of my hip movements. There is no big explosion, I tend to have two or three little eruptions. I respect a man who has the perseverance and skill to get me there.

Lisa, 19

game over. But, with multiples, there may be a building wave of orgasm where she has a small one and then allows you to continue. After a lull, she may have another small one and continue to have small ones until she's exhausted. In this case, there may be no final big bang. It's like a series of gentle waves rolling into a beach. For others, the experience is more like a tsunami – a few small waves of orgasm and then a lull, during which everything builds and builds and builds. This is a time when you are likely to get lockjaw – but don't ever stop unless asked. Without warning, a massive, bone-jarring tidal wave of sensation will come crashing down on your lover. Sure, she may be so sensitive afterwards that she throws you off the bed and curls up into a fetal position, but hell, what a thing to watch!

No orgasms

You will notice that, earlier on in the introduction to the orgasm section, I said every woman is physically capable of achieving an orgasm. That's the key: physically. If a mental issue causes some type of block, however, then her body won't react to its own physical signals and she may never orgasm. There are different degrees of difficulty in this scenario. Some women may be able to orgasm by themselves, but not with partners, while some women may not even be able to masturbate themselves to orgasm.

You reaction in this situation will depend on your lover. If it's a one night stand, then perhaps you will need to accept that you can not change her life overnight, that her lack of orgasm is no reflection on you, and that you enjoyed yourself anyhow.

With a relationship that is a little more serious, however, the lack of orgasm can become a horrible thing to confront. It's hard not to feel like it is your fault when your lover doesn't have an orgasm, but you will need to ask her advice on this issue. It could just be a lack of technique and you need to work a little harder. But, if she has issues in her past with abuse or with other painful sexual experiences, then she should consider some form of therapy.

There are baby steps any woman can take to help herself. If your lover can orgasm by herself, then would she let you listen outside her door? Or would she let you record it – even if it's just an old fashioned audio-only tape – so she can then "mail you an orgasm"? Can you get her started with foreplay and great muff-diving and then she finishes off? What about if she does her best job of faking it for you, like an Oscar-winning performance, just so she learns that it's nothing to be embarrassed or worried about in front of you? Get creative, and don't play the blame game.

I don't know why but, until you, I could never orgasm with a lover. Well, I do know why, but it's hard to deal with. I had an abusive childhood and, somewhere along the way, I picked up the idea that if I was always silent and non-responsive in my life, then I wouldn't be hit. When I'm alone, I can orgasm with no issue. Slowly though, you've been encouraging me to let go of myself in front of you. I think I laughed so hard when I emailed you a home video of myself that I started to realize it was something I could overcome. It's not easy, and I still have issues, but they are solvable.

Tracey, 35

Chapter 3: It's Not Just About the Pink Parts

You may be about ready to throw this book down now and get to it. After all, you've learned all about the anatomy of a woman. You've brushed up on your techniques. You've learned some new stuff you're willing to try and you can't wait to head down to the sex shop to buy some toys to assist. But slow down! Women are more than walking vaginas.

Sometimes, the hardest bit of oral sex isn't actually your technique or your lack of knowledge about anatomy. Sometimes, it's a lack of insight into the female mind that holds you back. But, given my years of experience with women from all cultures, I've got a firm grasp on exactly what you may need to know to succeed.

Really, negotiating oral sex is like negotiating any business arrangement. There will be objections. There will be timing issues. There will be gals that need a cost-benefit-analysis of the whole decision. So, you just need to learn to react like any sales person and have prepared responses to overcome objections. You may have to pitch your case. But aren't the results worth it??

Recognizing Your Situation

Going down on the one-night stand

You've met a girl – at a party, in a bar, online, whatever. You've got her to agree to have sex with you not long after you've just met. Is this situation a slam-dunk? No. When a girl agrees to casual sex, most of the time she is thinking about penetration-with-penis style sex--the old-fashioned stuff. She's horny and she wants to get off.

Since we're going to assume she doesn't know you, then there is a fair chance she won't be intending to let you go down on her. It could be seen as too intimate for a woman on a one-night stand – something she needs to be able to relax into.

The trick here is to realize that being horny is not the real, full story, even if the woman has convinced herself it is. She may have all sorts of other mind games secretly hidden too – wanting more than a one night stand perhaps, hoping you'll feel the same after a night in the sack, wanting company or intimacy. She could be bored, drunk, or feeling a little destructive and wanting to be out of control. There are a million different reasons she has agreed to go home with you. After all, if it was just a simple case of wanting an orgasm with no extra baggage, she would go home to her vibrator. The fact she has allowed a man into her bed means something else is going on. It will be your job to figure out what she wants or needs and then use this to convince her to let you go down on her!

Hopefully you did your groundwork when you picked her up. Do you know why she was out at the bar, party or surfing that web dating site? How has her week been prior to meeting you? Is she recently single? Stressed at work? Think really hard about the conversations topic you've shared. This may be your clue. If she is feeling lonely or wanting intimacy then the correct approach is not to think of a rough and ready one night stand. Think more of keeping the conversation flowing and lots of touching all over her body. Be a gentleman. Let her decide to surrender to you!

If she is angry over something or trying to erase an ex-boyfriend, then you can be extra manly in your approach. Let her know that you can make her cum so hard that

I've always been a dancing fiend. I love to go out and hit the clubs, in tight little mini-shorts and heels. And sure, sometimes I let guys pick me up – or I'll hunt for a guy that I want to pick up. On those occasions I really am thinking about sex, not oral sex. There is nothing worse than getting a would-be lover home who wants to go down on you – when I've got a case of Disco Crutch. I just know that I'm all sweaty and messy and it's not sexy. But if a guy can smoothly work his way into suggesting a shower – then I might change my mind. But only a solo shower. I don't want some guy I just met in my shower with me. I can almost hear the violins from Psycho screeching then. Truly though, there is nothing worse than Disco Crutch. No, I lie! Don't eat too many onions because then you'll discover something I call Onion Snatch.

Larissa, 22

she's going to forget about everything else in the universe. Tell her you are going to take on the workload for the night and position her on her back. Take control.

If the issues aren't obvious, you may just have to bide your time and let her raise the objections. Use any of the standard responses in the objections section to follow.

Going down and the fling

This is probably the best thing that can happen to a man: somehow you've convinced a girl to sleep with you more than once. Yet, it's not really a relationship. Maybe she's married, maybe you're married, and hey, no judgement there, but for whatever reason you have been having repeated encounters with the same woman with no permanent relationship in sight.

This, my friend, is the Holy Grail of cunnilingus. This is the one time in your life when you can throw every single

---

Want to increase your chance for Round 2?

Do
- Ask permission
- Compliment her body
- Go slow
- Make eye contact
- Learn to watch her body's reactions
- Get feedback
- Keep learning new things

Don't
- Keep changing styles in one session
- Push a suggestion too much
- Be upset if she doesn't orgasm
- Fall asleep/walk away immediately
- Keep score

---

one of the techniques, positions and toys at the woman and just watch what happens. She may not like it all; she may even hate some of it, but consider it your own private experiment. If you're in the middle of a hot affair, she'll probably be comfortable enough to let you know what she's thinking so you should almost be taking notes. For, when the fling ends – and all flings do end, either burning themselves out or going the opposite way and turning into something long term and committed – you will want to remember how it all went down, so to speak. And then you can take that experience and move on.

The key to successful oral sex in a fling is to start conversations with words like, "I was wondering if you'd like to try…." Or "Have you ever….", "What do you think about…." Be playful and suggestive and watch your woman blossom. Enjoy, I'm jealous already.

Going down long-term

So, maybe your fling ended in marriage or perhaps you decided to move in together. Or, maybe you married your high-school sweetheart. Somehow, you have found yourself in the situation where you are going to be looking at the same pussy for the foreseeable future. For this scenario, I'm going to rule out non-monogamy. If you are in an open relationship or going to cheat, then you have more options. However, let's assume you need assistance in the bedroom in a settled down, marriage-like situation. This is absolutely tough going. There probably a great chance that the oral sex has dwindled down to non-existence. This could be partly her fault or partly your fault, but it is going to be an uphill battle. Don't give up hope. In the right situation you can rekindle and keep those oral sex fires burning.

It all starts with housework. Yes, it sounds sexist, but no long-term partner is going to be able to relax into oral sex if her mind is tallying up all of the things she thinks you've done wrong. So, make an effort for a day or two to be wonderful with the chores and kids. Not just a few hours of effort – she'll see through that! Try a *real* effort for a few days. Then, try a glass of wine over dinner. Try a massage. Throw every seduction technique you have at her. Do not attempt to demand equal treatment--like a blow job. Then, work your way down her body. By now, she's probably in heaven, wondering where her perfect man came from. And you can play freely.

Setting the mood

- Ban the TV from the bedroom – or at least hide the PS3 or Wii.
- Have music on hand
- Be able to change lighting style – a dimmer or a few well positioned lamps will do
- Climate control – she won't starfish when it is too cold to take off her jacket
- Make the bed
- Keep the floor clutter free
- Make sure blinds are closed

In long term relationships, things can fall into a routine. So, you are going to have to break that routine. Book a hotel room. Clean the bedroom and make it look ready for sex and not just sleep with things such as nice new sheets and mood lighting.

You may think is all very unfair and far too much effort. But think back to your single days. How much effort did you put into seduction with your lovers? How many times did you head out looking for action before you finally got some? How much money did you spend on dinner dates? Probably a lot. A long-term relationship does not mean sex-on-tap and, even if you can get away with the odd bit of fast, routine sex, oral-sex-on-tap is never going to happen unless you continue the effort. You may face a million objections, so the section below will be a huge benefit.

Common Objections from Women

The whole thing is too embarrassing

This kind of objection usually comes from a woman who was not raised in any kind of sex positive household. She's embarrassed or uncomfortable with her own genitals. She may even be worried about the secretions her body makes or the noises she makes. Try to find out exactly what she means by embarrassing.

The only way to win in this situation is to convince her she is normal. Tell her that you know porn and magazines are usually

> Verse 7:2 in the King James Version of the Biblical **Song of Songs** appears to contain a direct reference to cunnilingus, although most English translators translate the key term as "naval". Probably goes down better in church that way. An alternate translation could read as follows: "Your vulva is a rounded crater, never lacking mixed wine."

airbrushed, that real women are different, and explain that you're experienced enough to make her feel comfortable. You can also reassure her that you will go slow and will turn the lights off if need be. This type of woman would not want mirrors anywhere near her either. You might want to use some music to cover any sounds that may freak her out as well.

I'm too smelly

Does she mean smelly right now, or smelly in general? If the answer is right now, then the solution is simple – a shower. Or even a wipe down with a clean, wet face towel. If she means smelly in general, she is probably in a similar situation to the embarrassed girl above whom doesn't like her own body. So, again, reassuring her that her smell is normal, that it's not fishy, and that you aren't repulsed will all help. If she really is smelly when you get there, then perhaps she does need a visit to a gynaecologist!

I've got my period

As discussed earlier, this can be a total brush off from a woman. Or it can mean that she is feeling a bit unsexy and gross. Again, a shower may help, plus a fresh tampon.

A Hell's Angel whose colors include red wings indicates that he or she has performed cunnilingus on a woman who was having her period at the time.

If she is a little more adventurous, a shower and then laying a towel underneath her bottom is probably enough because a woman doesn't gush blood. Just steer clear of penetration if you want to keep it clean. She may be much more sensitive or even in a bit of pain, so slow and gentle is the way to go.

I'm too sensitive

There isn't really any such thing as "too sensitive." It's another code word for being uncomfortable and not confident. If you have slept with this woman before, she may be trying to tell you that perhaps you are too rough. Maybe you are putting too much pressure on her clit or using your teeth. It could also mean "ticklish." You will have to ask her to explain exactly what she means when she uses this excuse.

I'm not fresh

"Fresh" is a word that the media and the tampon industry has forced on girls. These days, there is a panty liner for every day of the month if you want one – any secretion is deemed to be unladylike and likely to ruin your underwear. So, not being fresh could just be an inexperienced woman not knowing what secretions are normal. That is easy to fix. Your fingers should be able to feel what is normal and what isn't. You will just need to reassure her.

> The Foo Fighters track "All My Life" is about cunnilingus, this is mentioned by the lyrics "I love it, but I hate the taste".

Fresh can sometimes trick you though. A lot of my lovers used this excuse when they really meant to say, "I've just been to the toilet and now I'm afraid my pussy will smell like urine or that I may have cleaned myself wrong and even left bits of paper." A woman will never tell you she just peed when the topic of oral sex comes up because who wants to link the two concepts together? It is better to pretend they don't use the same parts of the anatomy for these two purposes! Again, the solution is the shower!

I'm too hairy

Hairy is in the mouth of the beholder really. What is too hairy for some of us is not nearly enough for others. So, the first line of attack for this objection is to let the woman know that you like hair. Perhaps ask to see just exactly what she means. This could get the foreplay going and she may even forget she ever objected. This is fine if you can cope with hair.

If you agree with her - that she actually is too hairy - then the sexiest, hottest thing in the universe is to offer to shave her. This will probably work on all objections for the fling, but perhaps not so much for the long-term partner who may find it a bit odd.

If you do get to wield the razor, then make sure you're sensible with it. Don't give the girl any reason to mistrust you. This means you shouldn't joke around or she may decide you are a razor-wielding-maniac and kick you to the curb.

The correct approach is to lather her up slowly, run your hands over her legs and thighs, perhaps even a little bit of play with your fingers. Then, drop to your knees with the razor and shave with the direction of the hair. Inward and upwards from the thighs toward her belly button is the general direction. If the issue is more thickness and curliness than an urban sprawl of hair, the best tool for the job are nail scissors. Pull the curls out gently and clip them quite short.

It feels too intense

This is similar to the objection about being sensitive. What she really may mean is that you are putting too much pressure directly on her clit. Or, maybe not you, but a past partner did so and it has scared her off. The clitoris and the clitoral hood are very delicate and the sensation can be far too much for some women. You are probably better off letting her know that you can change your technique to suit her and that she can tell you if you get it wrong! In that case, focus your efforts slightly around or below the clitoral area.

As soon I hear the words "too intense," I stop everything and then start again very slowly in a different spot. It seems to work for me. If I'm using my tongue tip, I'll switch right away to the tongue surface too.

I don't know you well enough

This is an objection for the one-night stand. It's probably a trust thing. Asking to perform oral sex on a woman puts her in the most vulnerable position possible. Anything could happen. She may have fears about being raped, stabbed, bitten, robbed or goodness knows what else. They've all heard horror stories from TV shows and even from watching the news.

You could suggest she sits on your face if that will make her feel safer. This may not work either, because she will still have her back to the room. You could suggest her place, or a nice hotel room, rather than your place. Or suggest leaving the lights on.

If it is not a trust thing, then the other possibility is that she feels it is far too intimate an act for a first meeting. This is where you need to show your charm – suggest that this is a perfect situation because she doesn't have to ever see you again. Therefore, she can totally let go of her inhibitions without having to worry about being embarrassed! It could be a chance to experiment…

I know you too well

If you've got a friend-turned-lover or are in a long-term relationship, this objection can sometimes be the hardest one to overcome. Maybe, once upon a time in your relationship, there used to be heaps of oral sex. But then it dwindled. Or maybe you're so used to drinking beer and hanging out as friends that, when it finally turned into a romp in the bedroom, things got awkward. Either way, the cause is the same. The woman doesn't feel comfortable being overly sexual in front of you. She's probably worried about your judgement or she's self-conscious.

The trick here is to make her think that oral sex is no big

deal. Take all of the sexiness out of it. Keep the lights on, put bad music on or even turn on the TV. Start things happening away from the bedroom. Stay half-dressed. Start a drinking contest or a tickle war. Be stupid and silly and see if you can release some of the self-consciousness. And then just try to "fall" into bed – it will be much easier once that tension is gone. You need to let the woman know that you can be silly and laugh during oral sex. And yet, it can still feel great!

"I hate the noises." Or "It's too noisy." Or "It's not noisy enough."

Women are hard characters to please. Why is noise such a common objection during oral sex? I think it's because a woman retreats into her head when she gets turned on and outside noises can make or break her mood.

Her first fear may be the slurping, sucking noises that can happen during good sex. That's an easy problem to solve – music! But then she may say it's "too noisy." This usually means that the noise in the background is distracting her from her rhythm. So, you'll need to turn off the music and TV and kick the cats out whatever it takes so she can work herself into a frenzy.

On the other end of the spectrum is the woman who is afraid of what is in her head. She doesn't like whatever she is thinking, so she wants background noise to bring her back into her own body. Again, you've no choice but to follow her instructions. Start an argument at this point and you're likely to be kicked out.

I look ugly down there or in that position

It doesn't matter what you say in this scenario. Trust me. If a woman says she feels ugly or that her female parts look ugly, then that will be enough to turn her off from sex. You can try and let her know she's normal, but you're best bet in this situation is to distract her. Suggest a different position. Tell her you'll wear a blindfold. Let her sit on your face, rather than be in any of the positions on her back. Promise her you'll keep your eyes closed! Or of course, turn out the lights!

I'll feel like I owe you one

You can admit to it. Men, and women too, are scorekeepers. Massages, breakfasts in bed, who took the trash out last, all of this enters our head and is tallied on a scorecard. Oral sex is renowned for this. How often have

I was married for 5 years before I started looking for satisfaction outside of the marital home. My husband was one of those sex bargainers. "I will give you a massage if you give me head" or "I will go down on you, only if we can try the 69er". I finally decided to post an ad online for some quality "me time". Luckily, you replied and taught me how real men treat a lady. You were gentle at first and never asked for anything in return. After a little time and a lot of coxing, I can admit I have never had such great sexual encounters. As for my husband, it was a deal breaker. I have moved on from you, but will always be thankful for the things you showed me.

Peta, 40

you gone down on a girl, only because you wanted a blow job? Or, after you got a blow job, you gave a half-hearted attempt to return the favor but turned in a poor performance? These things can kill you in a fling or a long-term relationship. If you offer a girl oral sex, it's best that you expect nothing in return. Or else she may think she can't be bothered with it if, at the end, she's expected to service you or if she thinks next time you'll be expecting her to perform for you as a payback.

You will need to totally let go of those expectations. Give oral sex freely, without payback needed, and you'll find the women much more receptive of it at any time!

What if you kiss me afterwards?

Most women are repulsed by the idea of tasting themselves. They do not want to be kissed after your mouth has been on their vaginas. They don't want you to stop mid-act and come up for a kiss either. It can make them squirm – and not in a good way. They may be so stressed about what will happen afterwards that they'll stop the whole show. Don't let this happen. If you've made the mistake in the past, admit it and tell her in future you'll be more considerate. If she raises the concern or says something about a past lover's habits, tell her flat out that you would never do the same without asking permission.

I'm too dry

Dryness does not mean your woman is not aroused. Dryness can be a medical condition. In that case, you may have to use lubricant for her to enjoy oral sex. You may need to experiment with one that tastes okay to you.

Dryness can also mean there hasn't been enough foreplay. Oral sex shouldn't necessarily be considered a first step in foreplay that you take along the way to penetration. In fact, it can be the final act. So, if you hear this excuse, then what the gal may really mean is, "You are moving too fast. Slow down."

If you think your lover will appreciate dirty talking, making a comment about helping to get her wet would probably work at this stage.

I just don't like it

If a woman says this, it usually means she has had some bad experiences in the past. There are two ways around this. The first, if you are confident in your technique, is to bravely state that she hasn't had you before. Take control, gauge her responses and change her mind. This works best on the one night stand or fling. The safer option is to let her be your teacher. Ask her what she doesn't like about it. Hopefully, it will fall into one of the above categories. Otherwise, suggest that she talk you through every step and get feedback along the way. It keeps her in control, gives her what she wants and allows the use of dirty talk. This approach, if discussed first, is the quickest and easiest way to give her the best orgasm possible and change her mind.

Common Issues the Ladies Think We Have

We're too soft or too sloppy

This complaint tends to come from women who are frustrated with your performance. They're probably bored out of their minds. There is nothing more annoying for a woman then to agree to some hot sex, only to find it limp and soggy.

Soft or sloppy oral sex is a sign of bad technique or lack of confidence in what it is you're supposed to be doing. You don't need to be drooling like some monster from Alien all over the woman and you don't need to be licking or nibbling like it's a gourmet ice cream. You need to be firm and assured in your strokes, and there is nothing unmanly about asking her just how she likes it.

"My very first time someone went down on me was when I was 15. I hadn't had sex yet and, through my youthful wisdom of alcohol, a begging boyfriend and the thoughts that at least I couldn't get pregnant, I agreed. It was the worst thing I had experienced. There was no lead up to the event, his tongue was suddenly everywhere, teeth somehow got involved and it was like he forgot that it was about me too. It was like a little puppy finding his first chew toy. It took 3 years and 2 more relationships until I finally let you show me how it was meant to be. I have never looked back and am more then happy to show all the puppies out there how to control themselves!!"

Nessa, 26

We suck too hard or graze with our teeth

At the other end of the complaint spectrum is the issue of sucking too hard or using teeth. These methods should be banned from the bedroom, unless you are in a long-term relationship and have already had a conversation with the lady and she has specifically told you that she prefers it rough. That would be a rare lady, indeed! Otherwise, never let your teeth out to play and don't try to pull the clitoris into your mouth or suck it like a boiled lolly.

The porn problem

Some of us think there is nothing wrong with extra excitement in the bedroom, such as going down with your fave porn in the background. It gives you something to listen to or even to watch while your tongue does the workout. WRONG. It's too much multi-tasking and most women would find it distracting, if not downright rude. They want to feel like they are the center of your attention!

Talking dirty

Most women will have a preferred word for their genitals. They may also have words that they hate and would never respond to. As a guideline, steer clear of the word cunt in your dirty talking. Even pussy can be a huge turn off to some women. It's best to listen to them talk about themselves, if you can, and then repeat the words they use.

Full frontal

You do not need to put a vagina on like a snorkel and attempt to breathe through it. Plunging your full face into the nether regions will likely cause discomfort, if not disgust. The aim is not to get your hair wet or to suffocate. Concentrate on where the nerve endings are – at the clitoris and the first inch or so of the vagina. Sometimes, this method is used in an attempt to cover up a general lack of knowledge. But, after reading the techniques part of this book, there should be no excuse for that, should there!?

Not settling on one method

The basic rule should be that if a woman is enjoying what you do, either demonstrating this by groaning, or a slight bucking of hips, then don't change it. You don't need to prove your mastery of technique by changing your movements every few seconds. This will not allow a girl to reach orgasm, and she'll probably grab you by your hair or ears and attempt to keep you in the one position. Most women need a slow and steady, consistent movement. This becomes more important the closer to orgasm she is. Changing your style as her moans become louder could stop her entirely.

If you want to experiment, then try one new technique each time you go down on her. Don't try 76 techniques in two minutes.

We don't enjoy it

There is nothing worse than a facial expression of distaste about the whole going down experience. If you don't enjoy it, then you need to figure out why. If it's the taste and smell of a normal gal that you don't like, then you may have to experiment with flavored lubes or even dental dams. Or, you might want to stick to going down only while she's in the shower.

If you can't mask your distaste, then you'll have to fake it like an Oscar winning actor until the lights go out. Then, you can relax as you perform in the dark! I am not here to judge you. If you truly, truly cannot stand the act, and reading this book hasn't changed your mind and you can't hide this fact from your lover, then you really need to fess up! At least tell her how you feel. She needs to know so she can decide how important this fact is to her and her own sexual satisfaction.

If you continue to go down on your lover, but she knows you don't like it, then not only are you ruining it for her, you may be damaging her long term enjoyment and she may carry insecurities to another lover.

Using your tongue as a dart

A clitoris is not a dartboard and your tongue should not be used like a weapon. Zeroing in on her clitoris and making a stabbing motion quickly will not win you any points in the bedroom. In the worse case scenario, this may hurt. More likely, however, she will think you are a fool. She may also wonder if you have issues about her taste or smell if you are attempting to keep you face free of the area…

Relax your tongue and use it to its full potential.

Keeping score

This was listed in the objections women have and I just thought I should reiterate it here. There is nothing worse than making it known that you are only performing cunnilingus so you can score a blow job, or some other sexual favor. Ditch the score card.

Lockjaw or tired tongue

This happens to the best of us. You've read the techniques and everything is going well – until your tongue starts to get tired or your jaw aches. Really, you will need to just suck it up at this point and keep going. It would be cruel to stop. For an aching tongue, try moving your face closer to her clitoris so your tongue doesn't have to reach as far. This should keep your mouth from drying out and should prevent your tongue from getting sore from stretching over your teeth. For a sore jaw, you need to relax your position. Don't try and "lock" it in place – this is why is gets sore in the first place. Besides, you do not need to have your mouth open that wide. You could also try stretching exercises with your mouth before hand and in private. Pretend you are yawning and move your jaw from side to side. Massage it a little. Now get in there boy, and have fun!

Chapter 4: Going Beyond

Congratulations! If you've made it this far into the book, you are in for a treat. By now, you've learned some techniques. You've got the anatomy sorted. You've learned how to overcome any objections that a woman raises and you've figured out what she really means when she tries to communicate. So it's time to take all of those skills on the road for a great adventure. Let's think about all of the ways you can apply these new talents. The topics raised below are fairly outrageous. They're the stuff of legend. These are the things that give you bragging rights with your buddies.

Anilingus

It's a horrid sounding term, with a horrid reputation...but it really shouldn't be that way! It refers, of course, to playing with your lover's butt. This is an advanced area to venture into because most women have firm views on if they are "up the butt" girls or not and no amount of persuasion can change the mind of a firmly conservative lover. Hence, there has been no mention of this erotic zone earlier in the book.

If you do have a lover who is open-minded, then there are many things you can do to increase her pleasure in oral sex. You can use your tongue on that area too – rimming is the art of rolling your tongue around the entrance to the anus. Yes, this can be seen as a gay boy practice, but you are man enough not to care about that, right? It feels good for the woman. You can also try licking the area from her anus up to her vagina.

When playing with penetration with you fingers, you can try a lubed finger in her butt, either alone or with another finger in her vagina too. Just don't switch fingers around or you may introduce bowel nasties to her vagina and that isn't cool.

You can also use sex toys, such as anal plugs along with vibrators on her clit or a dildo in her vagina. Just make sure anything you insert into her anus has a flared base and is designed for anal play–otherwise it can be sucked inside her and you will have to spend the night in ER.

Once I had a lover who was crazy for butt play. She sometimes would forget about the safety basics and want to put her vibrator in her butt – and I would have to stop her. In my experience, if you want to experiment in this area, go and buy a toy together! It's great foreplay.

If you are thinking about butt play, then hygiene will be your main concern. Make sure she doesn't feel the need to poo before you start your butt play. That feeling means there are feces quite close to being expelled and your finger or anal toy may encounter some. Your lover may not have considered shaving or waxing that area either, so there may be a fair amount of hair. This can hold all sorts of unsexy things so, if it is a worry, then a thorough shower will sort it out. This is not the sexy, gentle, fun, together shower, but really a solo shower she needs to have to really scrub herself or to squat and shave right up her crack. It's not normally an erotic preparation.

By now, you've probably got the idea that you can't just spring anal play onto your lover while in the middle of oral sex. That's also why it's an advanced thing. You will have to negotiate the situation and pick a moment that is right for the woman so she has time to prepare. Then play away! Going down on a woman while penetrating her can make her orgasm in spectacular ways, which certainly makes it worth the effort.

Threesomes

Let's use your imagination now and put you in a situation where you have not only one woman, but two. That's two vaginas to play with. What exactly can you do in this situation? In an ideal world, at least one of the women will be bisexual because this will increase the possibilities for fun.

One night my boyfriend and I went to a swinger's club with another couple. I had been with girls in the past and was happy about the whole idea. We did try to both go down at the same time on one woman we both thought was hot. It was a bit of a shambles really – sharing a clit is hard work and your shoulders kinda bump and get in the way. Still it was a pretty amazing experience.

Ellen, 27

So, you could go down on one woman, while the other woman straddles her face. Or one of the women and you can both go down on the other woman. This will require some co-ordination. Just like in a game of doubles tennis, when you can only work your side of the court and need to call for the ball, in this type of oral sex, you really need to stick to one side! Otherwise, it can be too crowded. In this case, one of you can surface and get to work on the nipples or other erogenous zones.

Another way of enjoying this is to have one girl propped up on cushions with the other girl going down on her. And then you can have sex with that girl in the doggy style position. Then, you get to watch the oral sex while having your own penetrative sex. Fun for all involved! You will need to get everyone positioned quite carefully; otherwise

I gotta tell you, sleeping with a married couple isn't always a good idea. I'm a bi girl, maybe even leaning a bit more toward women, and I met this great couple online. We went out for dinner – pizza and beer at a very hip place. They had a babysitter back home for their young son. It all seemed so surreal and normal all at the same time. We then went back to my place. I was going down on the wife and the husband was trying to fuck me from behind. That way he could make eye contact with his wife and I was just the "conduit" in the middle. Nice idea, right? Except the wife started go off! Yelling things along the lines of, "This is the best oral sex of my life!". It got to the point where I felt a bit sorry for the husband. He was trying to please her in their married life, but obviously I was doing it better. He lost his hard-on. Then the wife realized she'd probably sounded a bit cruel, or ungrateful, so we stopped and spent the next half an hour trying to pay attention to him, and get his hard on back, but it was over.

Tegan, 23

the bed won't be long enough for all three bodies! You could always try standing at the end of the bed while the two women take up most of the bed's actual space.

Partner Swapping

You can always head to a sex club, or a partner swapping night, or arrange your own swapping over the Internet. In this scenario, you and another man would swap lovers. It would be up to you to decide if you want to stay in the same room or have the new lover all to yourself, but you may have to negotiate this.Having both couples in the same room may add extra excitement because you'll be able to watch your lover have oral sex. But, if she goes off into another room, then you may be able to experiment wildly with your new lover without worrying about her judgement. Either way, swapping is a great way to try something new. In these situations, make sure you having some code words worked out or ground rules for both couples so that everyone remains safe and comfortable. And don't forget to consider protection.

Hooking Up With Her Best Friend

What could be hotter than getting your lover to go down on another woman while you are there!? You can share parts of this book with her if she's worried about technique. I bet she isn't though – she's a girl, she owns her own set of female stuff, and probably has a million ideas she's like to try on another chick. The issue is going to be her own sexuality. If she is 100% totally, forever more and not-a-word-of-a-lie straight, then I don't like your chances of convincing her to try this advanced bit of oral sex fun. What you need is a girl that is a little bit flexible. You don't want say, a dyke that just hasn't come out yet, because chances are she'll run off with the other girl and leave you all alone. You want a lover from the grey area in between, and these days they aren't so hard to find. Some girls were gay-till-graduation types that had a college girlfriend before heading back to men. Some are pretty straight but, with a few drinks and some encouragement, are open to experiment. Some girls are pure bisexual creatures, with no preference either way. A bit of talk about past lovers and fantasies will tell you where on the scale your lover is.

If you do have a lover who is ready for this type of fun, then make sure you let her pick the other girl. She needs to be totally comfortable with the situation and the tension has to be between the women. Even if you aren't attracted to her choice, chances are you aren't going to give a damn when you have your pecker in your hand, watching you own live porn show take place in your own bed!

Don't try and force yourself into this situation either. Start as just the enthusiastic cheerleader on the sidelines and let the girls decide your involvement.

One last word of advice: be a bit careful about the other woman you bring into the circle. If it's secretly someone you like more than your current lover, then you're setting the scene for a nasty showdown. You may end up with no lovers because the two women will bond over their oral sex experience and probably gossip about you behind your back anyhow – so hitting on the other woman would, of course, not go unreported!

Multiple Partners

I just thought I should put a word of warning into this advanced section for those of you are contemplating leaving your long-term lover for someone newer or more enthusiastic about the idea of oral sex. As I've said before, I would never judge anyone. But, if you do decide to cheat, then the chances are you are going to learn more tricks or different ways of using the techniques mentioned in this book. You'll experiment more. The problem with this is that you may give yourself away back home. If you've only performed oral sex while your partner is on her back and suddenly you're wanting her on your face and you're spelling the alphabet rather than your old-school method, your lover may get suspicious.

Female Genital Mutilation

You may think that, in a book on sex, mentioning any of the "darker" sides would be a real mood killer. But this is the advanced section and these are advanced issues we are dealing with.

I'll put this into a scenario for you. You're out at a bar. You get talking to an exotic creature over a cocktail. She's a doctor and just finished her training. She's thinking about heading back home to Mali or Sudan to share what she has learned. She's up for an adventure – and she's picked you.

Back home, she tells you that she's been "circumcised". Why is this such a big deal? Well, it could mean any number of things. She could have had her clitoral hood removed, even her clitoris. She may have had her inner lips trimmed or removed. She may even have had her outer lips sewed shut, leaving only a small hole to allow urine and menstrual blood to pass. These practices are now usually referred to as Female Genital Mutilation or Female Genital Cutting. No doubt about it, it's a horrid practice. But, it is used in many African countries and in some Middle Eastern countries for a variety of cultural reasons.

This is uncharted territory for the average male and, if you find yourself in this situation, you are going to have to act emphatically. Listen to her story. If she does allow you to perform oral sex, then be very gentle. Ask questions to determine the extent of her injuries. She may not be able to orgasm, so don't place any pressure on her.

Artificial Vaginas (Vaginoplasty)

Okay, let's go back to the exotic scenario above. You see a lovely creature in the bar. She's tall, graceful, slender of hip. You cannot wait to take this supermodel home. At some stage, it is revealed to you that she is actually a post-operative transgender. Yes, once she was a he. But, after many a trip to the surgeon, she is now in possession of breasts, a new name, and an artificially created vagina.

Now, I've been in this situation. And I'll tell you one thing, if you think this makes me less of a man, or even gay or some such nonsense, then you really shouldn't be reading this advanced section. Some folk are born with the wrong bodies. Some are lucky enough to be able to afford to rectify the situation and there is nothing remotely homosexual about someone willing to cut off their own penis to feel more like the woman they are sure they are inside.

Of course, I was curious and my lovely supermodel was all too happy to educate me. In the end, there is nothing truly different to worry about. These gorgeous women can still reach orgasm and experience penetration. They will even look exactly like a real woman externally. Surgeons can do a remarkable job creating a vagina and clitoris – even the lips will look natural enough. Perhaps a little more innie than outie in most cases but, chances are that you may never have found out if you hadn't been told. The only thing to worry about is lubrication – you may need to use lube if the vagina is not self-lubricating. That will depend on the type of surgery your wonderful lover has had!

Heightening Sensation

If plain ol' vanilla oral sex is starting to get a bit boring, you could always try and experiment with heightening the sensations. Blindfolds, total silence – anything that removes one sense from the equation may heighten the feelings from oral sex, especially for the woman. You can use these types of techniques in a very romantic way – especially if you're talking about silk restraints and blindfolds. Or you can use these ideas in more a role-playing kind of way. These are things that would all need to be negotiated and are probably best left to the fling or the long-term relationship. Always make sure you have a "safe word." A safe word is a word or phrase that cannot be mistaken for normal sexual conversation. So the words, "stop, no, no more" should not be safe words. Try a silly word like pancake or banana or something similar. That way, if the role-playing is too much or if your lover wants out of her blindfold, she can use that word and you know that she needs you to stop immediately.

Chapter 5: The Happy Ending

So, what about me?

Now men, or at least, one man (which is *you* dear reader) has evolved and conquered the skills needed to hunt, gather, explore, romance, and, finally, to please a women in a way she can admit she wants. Now you ask, so, what about me? It is satisfying knowing that you have the moves, that you can make a woman squirm, scream and tremble with your wicked tongue. And you can't deny that, aimed with the right tools, you can help women overcome their inner worries and let them be free to enjoy one of the most intimate and exhilarating sexual acts. But still, you are left with a massive hunger for some of your own satisfaction. And why shouldn't a girl want to do all of this for you?

Well this is where it all comes together. You need to consider the skill you've learned and the possible payoffs. These payoffs were mentioned throughout the book, but are worth repeating.

One night stand

As discussed, for whatever horny, alcohol-induced reason, you have scored yourself that hot girl from the bar. This is the time to experiment with your new moves and fine-tune your techniques for use at later dates. If you embarrass yourself or don't quite get it right, you will just become a funny story that she will tell at her next girls' night out. On the other hand, if you pull out the moves and treat her right, your one night stand could turn into a fling. And you can't ask for more than that – sex and experimentation with no strings attached.

Fling

So we have decided that you are not going to use a score card. But, of all the women I have been with, if you please them, they *want* to please you. You might not get sex on this occasion but, when it is your turn, they will turn up the tricks for you. Remember, this is a time when both people can experiment the most and, by trying to please the women, when they have their turn, you can ask them for a few new things too.

Long term

All is not lost when you get lured into the sex only on special occasions style of relationship. By adding these new steps, slowly, into a relationship, your sex life is only going to improve. Again, if you never expect or ask for reciprocation, you will get it the most. Suddenly, your bored housewife will turn back into that foxy minx your first met. She will feel a more intimate bond and, at the very least, this will help increase the number or times you have sex. Also, by being selfless in the bedroom, she will start to overlook the fact you are somewhat lacking in the housework department.

Also from Secret Life Publishing:

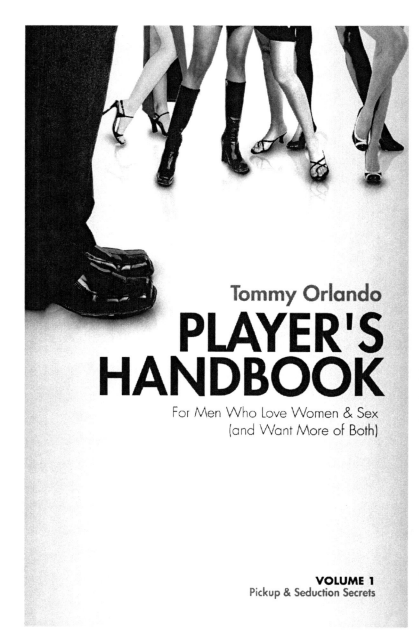

Tommy Orlando
PLAYER'S
HANDBOOK
For Men Who Love Women & Sex
(and Want More of Both)

VOLUME 1
Pickup & Seduction Secrets

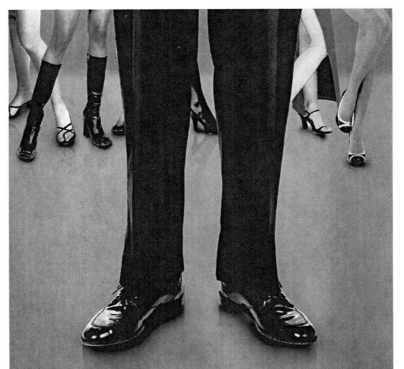

Tommy Orlando

PLAYER'S HANDBOOK

For Men Who Love Women & Sex
(and Want More of Both)

VOLUME 2
Advanced Pickup &
Seduction Secrets

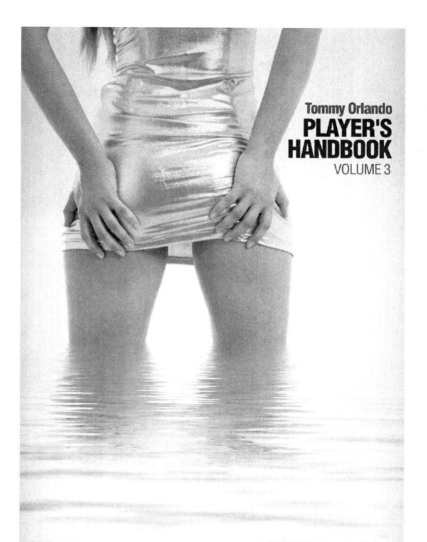

Tommy Orlando
PLAYER'S
HANDBOOK
VOLUME 3

MAKE HER SQUIRT!
A QUICK AND DIRTY GUIDE
TO FEMALE EJACULATION AND EXTENDED ORGASM

Tommy Orlando

PLAYER'S
HANDBOOK
VOLUME 4

WHAT TO EAT
(AND HOW TO EAT IT)
A QUICK AND DIRTY GUIDE
TO GIVING GREAT ORAL SEX

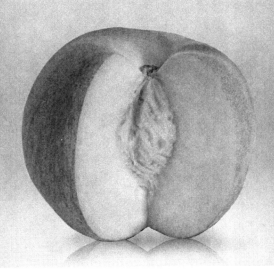

LaVergne, TN USA
28 April 2010
180855LV00001B/34/P